Intermittent Fasting for Women:

7 Simple Steps to Understanding & Mastering the Art of Intermittent Fasting for Women in Every Day Life!

Table of Contents

Intermittent Fasting for Women: 1
Table of Contents 2
Introduction 9
Chapter 1: Understanding Intermittent Fasting . 14

   What is Intermittent Fasting?
   Origins: Where Did Intermittent Fasting Come From?

      Intermittent Fasting Tip: Apple Cider Vinegar

   The Science of Intermittent Fasting: How Does It Work?

      Intermittent Fasting Tip: Fasting Is Habit & Determination, Not A Miracle Cure

   Why Try Intermittent Fasting?

      Intermittent Fasting Tip: Keep It Up!

Chapter 2: Intermittent Fasting for Women & Choosing the Right Plan for You 36

   Intermittent Fasting & The Female Form
   How Does Intermittent Fasting Benefit Women?
   How Is Intermittent Fasting Riskier for Women?
   Step One: Making A Plan That Will Get Results

Gather All the Information You Can
Determine Your Motivation & Set Realistic Goals
Asking the Right Questions
The Importance of Designing A Realistic Fasting Plan for Your Lifestyle
Intermittent Fasting Tip: The Best First Step Is the Baby Step

From Method to Mastering: The Different Types of Intermittent Fasting

The 16/8 Method: A Popular Choice for Busy Adults & Beginners
Alternate Your Fasting Schedule or Fast Every Other Day: A Universally Balanced Method of Intermittent Fasting
An Ideal Option for Women of All Ages: The 5/2 Intermittent Fasting Plan

Chapter 3: Setting Yourself Up for Success 64

Step Two: Be Prepared Before You Jump Right In!

Plan Your Exercise Based on How Your Body Feels
Intermittent Fasting Tip: Keep a Record of Your Personal Experience
Stock Your Kitchen to Support an Intermittent Fasting Routine
Intermittent Fasting Tip: Sometimes the Gradual Path Is the Best Path to Take
Get A Professional Opinion to Guarantee Health & Safety

Step Three: Schedule Your First Fasting Plan . 77

    Plan Out More Than Just One Week at A Time
    Choosing the Best Day to Start A New Intermittent Fasting Routine
    What to Expect in the First Week on a New Intermittent Fasting Schedule
    Intermittent Fasting Tip: Drink More Water Than You Were Before You Started Fasting

Chapter 4: Taking Your First Intermittent Fasting Steps 85

    Step Four: You Have a Plan... Now Take the Plunge!

        In the Days Before Your First Fasting Window
        Intermittent Fasting Tip: Don't Start A New Diet the Same Day You Start A New Fasting Schedule

    First Two Weeks Sample Intermittent Fasting Schedule for Women: The 5/2 Method

        Fasting Day One: Your First Fast & How to Go About It On the 5/2 Intermittent Fasting Method
        Feeding Days Two & Three: Back to Regular Calorie Consumption & Ready for Your Next Fast

Intermittent Fasting Tip: Listen to Your Mind & Body Throughout the Course of the Week

Fasting Day Four: Your Second Fasting Window & The Last One of the First Week

Feeding Days Five, Six & Seven: Relax, Reflect & Refuel Before the Start of Your Second Week

Fasting Day Eight: One More Hill, Then Nothing but Easy Valleys!

Feeding Days Nine & Ten: Keeping an Eye Out for the Subtle Effects

Fasting Day Eleven: Your Fourth Fasting Window & It's Feeling Like Second Nature by Now

Feeding Days Twelve, Thirteen & Fourteen: How Far You've Come & Where to Go from Here

Tips & Tricks for Conquering the First Two Weeks of Intermittent Fasting

Chapter 5: The Two Week Check-In Point & How It Can Make All the Difference In Successful Intermittent Fasting Plans 105

Chapter 6: Enjoying Your New Lifestyle Bolstered by Intermittent Fasting! 118

Conclusion 131

© Copyright 2018 by Chantel Stephens - All rights reserved.

The follow Book is reproduced below with the goal of providing information that is as accurate and reliable as possible. Regardless, purchasing this Book can be seen as consent to the fact that both the publisher and the author of this book are in no way experts on the topics discussed within and that any recommendations or suggestions that are made herein are for entertainment purposes only. Professionals should be consulted as needed prior to undertaking any of the action endorsed herein.

This declaration is deemed fair and valid by both the American Bar Association and the Committee of Publishers Association and is legally binding throughout the United States. Furthermore, the transmission, duplication or reproduction of any of the following work including specific information will be

considered an illegal act irrespective of if it is done electronically or in print. This extends to creating a secondary or tertiary copy of the work or a recorded copy and is only allowed with express written consent from the Publisher. All additional right reserved.
The information in the following pages is broadly considered to be a truthful and accurate account of facts and as such any inattention, use or misuse of the information in question by the reader will render any resulting actions solely under their purview. There are no scenarios in which the publisher or the original author of this work can be in any fashion deemed liable for any hardship or damages that may befall them after undertaking information described herein. Additionally, the information in the following pages is intended only for informational purposes and should thus be thought of as universal. As befitting its nature, it is presented without assurance regarding its

prolonged validity or interim quality. Trademarks that are mentioned are done without written consent and can in no way be considered an endorsement from the trademark holder.

Introduction

Intermittent Fasting has been taking the health and fitness world by storm for decades. A practice as old as the human species and the survival instincts that helped develop us into the strong, healthy individuals of today. All over the world, people following all kinds of diets and all kinds of lifestyles are weaving fasting windows into their daily lives to help improve their physical and mental health and wellness progression.

Congratulations on purchasing *Intermittent Fasting for Women: 7 Simple Steps to Understanding & Mastering the Art of Intermittent Fasting for Women in Every Day Life!* and thank you for joining those already benefiting from the advice and information provided in our succinct and educational guide. In doing so, you have taken the first step to designing, beginning and maintaining an effective Intermittent Fasting schedule.

This guide has been specifically created for women interested in Intermittent Fasting as a health and wellness tool to assist with reaching their personal health goals. The following chapters will cover not only the basics of Intermittent Fasting as a means of weight loss and health enhancement, but they will also cover topics such as:

- How to design a personalized Intermittent Fasting plan that fits your daily schedule
- The risks and benefits women particularly face more frequently when adding Intermittent Fasting to their regular lifestyle
- Practical tips and tricks for how to master Intermittent Fasting as a health and wellness practice
- How to maximize your fat burning processes with supplemental diets and fitness programs that work well when

used in pairing with Intermittent Fasting
- Next steps new and experienced Intermittent Fasting participants can take once their bodies have adjusted in order to further challenge their physical, mental and emotional selves, getting the most out of their Intermittent Fasting plans

With *Intermittent Fasting or Women: 7 Simple Steps for Understanding & Mastering the Art of Intermittent Fasting*, readers are not just getting a book full of information, they are also getting a pre-planned two-week intermittent fasting plan designed using the method most recommended for female fasters and for beginners to Intermittent Fasting as a health and wellness tool.

By the end of the guide, readers will feel more comfortable with the concept of Intermittent Fasting and all that defines it so they can take their first steps with confidence and take advantage of all the benefits the program has to offer. Even though women need to take greater care when preparing their Intermittent Fasting routines than men do, there is an abundance of positive health benefits women can gain from the right fasting schedule. Keep this book at your side throughout your Intermittent Fasting journey as a friend, a supporter, a guide and a quick reference when questions arise, or changes need to be made to your personal fasting schedule in order to maximize benefits or eliminate negative side effects.

There is no shortage of Intermittent Fasting books on the market and no limit of information available anywhere from social media to health and wellness community boards. Thanks for choosing *Intermittent Fasting for Women: 7 Simple Steps to Understanding & Mastering the Art of*

Intermittent Fasting! Packed with useful and valuable information from cover to cover, *Intermittent Fasting for Women* is a strong planning and preparation tool for women interested in starting their first Intermittent Fasting plan.

We hope you enjoy our guide and wish you ever bit of luck on your personal health journey. The main goal of this guide is to be helpful in getting you to your best physical, mental and emotional health with a strong and solid Intermittent Fasting routine personalized to help you meet your goals!

Chapter 1: Understanding Intermittent Fasting

In a society flooded with miracle remedies, all-natural diets, and rotating fitness trends, it can be easy to get lost when seeking the answers or guidance you need. Information is critical to get started with the right options to improve your health, boost your energy and feel better in general. While choosing one specific path works for some, most people end up blending and adjusting fitness and dieting programs that support one another to meet their unique health needs and goals.

Intermittent Fasting is one such option that has gained a global following as one of the most successful modern health and fitness programs on the market. This is particularly true for those looking to lose weight, build muscle or take advantage of the numerous other physical, mental and emotional benefits that fasting can offer. Medical experts, dieticians, and nutritionists have spent years promoting Intermittent Fasting as a form of treatment or effective supplemental wellbeing program for a variety of medical and health concerns.

What is Intermittent Fasting?

Fasting is the act of ceasing normal daily food consumption (or severely reducing calorie intake) for a set of fasting and eating windows designed to achieve a certain goal. It is a widely respected practice with centuries of evidence to support its effectiveness and benefits for improving one's physical and mental wellbeing.

It is still regularly performed around the world for any number of personal reasons:

- Some religions use fasting as a means of penance or as an act of devotion

- There are endless health and medical uses for fasting ranging from weight loss to lowering blood sugar levels in diabetic patients
- In extreme cases, fasting can be used as a means of survival to save rations when food is scarce

With as much support and positive buzz swirling around health and fitness communities, there is still hesitation in promoting and joining in on intentional fasting despite its long-standing reputation and many health benefits. This is no wonder considering most people have learned throughout their childhood and in health classes at school about the importance of partaking in at least three full meals a day. Nutrition is fundamental in maintaining a healthy lifestyle and skipping meals can have damaging effects on the body and mind including:

- **Increased Risk of Developing an Eating Disorder:** Unplanned fasting, or intentionally not eating without a set health strategy, can quickly and dangerously evolve into bulimia or anorexia. The reason for this is that avoiding food consumption and forcing oneself not to eat on a regular basis can develop into a psychological effect often not considered when weighing the risks of fasting as a weight loss tool.
  - Many people are confused at what the difference is between fasting and having an eating disorder. Fasting is a controlled restriction of calorie consumption that is safely planned and executed in order to reach a predetermined health goal. Eating disorders are compulsive psychological

disorders built off of starvation as a weight loss plan.
- Sometimes these disorders are brought on by skipping a few meals as a time, which develops into a habit. In some cases, eating disorders are initiated by emotional concerns or hormonal imbalances.

- **Loss of Energy & Decreased Performance:** Recklessly skipping meals takes a toll on the mind, as well as the body. A sudden drop in glucose (the brain's main fuel source, which mostly comes from consumed carbohydrates) is one of the first physical effects felt by fasters. Without the regular glucose levels, and with little else being produced to replace it in the early days, those new to fasting notice they are not as focused, have less muscle strength and stamina and are constantly fighting fatigue.

- **Fluctuations in Blood Pressure & Sugar:** For people with blood related conditions such as hypertension and diabetes, fasting is still an option. It's all about finding a way to balance food consumption with the body's natural processes. One of the benefits of Intermittent Fasting is that it can be used to successfully lower blood sugar and blood pressure levels in those who suffer from related conditions. However, if not monitored or done without the appropriate preparation, it can have dangerous results.

However, when used properly and effectively monitored, the positive effects of Intermittent Fasting can make all the difference for some people's overall health. In order to combat the potential negative side effects, fasting can mean completely avoiding food for some, while others fast by strictly decreasing the number of calories they consume during fasting times. It all comes down to the individual's needs and how their body reacts to regular fasting.

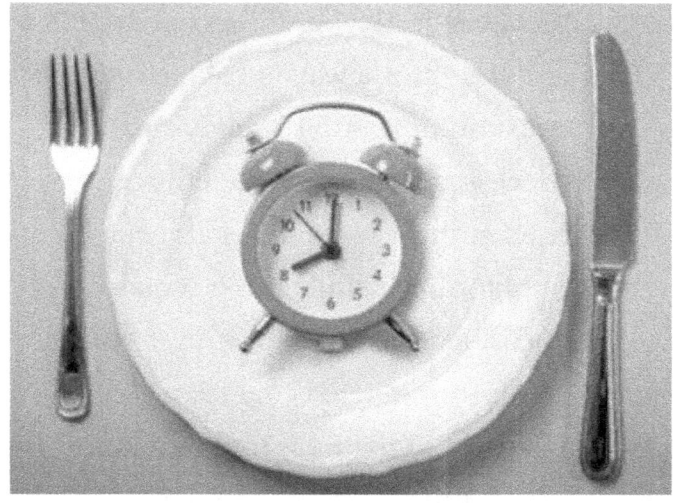

In most instances, this unwillingness or reluctance to start fasting comes from not having enough information or the right information about how it is being utilized as a powerful weight loss option. The goal of this guide is to expand your knowledge by providing all of the information you could ever need about Intermittent Fasting! The seven simple steps weaved throughout the guide will assist you in designing an Intermittent Fasting schedule that works for you based on individual needs, personal health goals, current health status, and existing conditions. Before getting to the first steps, let's take a closer look at the fundamentals of Intermittent Fasting.

Origins: Where Did Intermittent Fasting Come From?

Fasting has been a natural part of life in one form or another since the origins of humankind. At its most basic level, fasting is a survival tool developed by early humans as a way to survive during long periods without food such as deep winter when many animals are in hibernation or after natural disasters such as plagues or floods when crops were unexpectedly destroyed. Instead of just giving into starvation or going straight to uprooting their community in search of more bountiful lands, they learned to restrict their calorie intake and ration their food to only consume enough to survive and make their reserves last until conditions improved.

Apart from survival, in countries and cultures across the planet, fasting is often most commonly associated with religious practice, devotion and ceremony. Long-standing religions with the most ancient roots are best known for this and incorporate a form of fasting into their beliefs.

Muslims of the Islamic belief fast during the holy month of Ramadan as a way of displaying their devotion to their beliefs for all to see. This form of fasting is more absolute than those used for medical and dieting purposes, eliminating even their water and liquid consumption during their 12-hour daily fasting windows (sunrise to sunset) and continuing their daily food consumption at night. Practitioners are free to eat normally within the dietary restrictions of Islam during eating windows and throughout the rest of the year.

- Due to the risk of serious digestive distress, potentially life-threatening dehydration and metabolic issues associated with increased calorie consumption during the evening hours just before bed, this form of fasting is not recommended for those using it as a means of improving their overall strength and wellness.

Christians are not required to fast for their religion but have used fasting for centuries as a means of getting closer to God. The practice is believed to prove an individual worshipper's true dedication, serve as a proper act of penance and strengthen their personal commitment through sacrifice and self-control. Forty days is the standard amount of time for experienced fasters, but some will fast on the holy day of Sunday while others will fast throughout the Catholic celebration of Lent.

Buddhism is another belief system famous for fasting as a form of devotion and discipline. Buddhism promotes a consistent form of Intermittent Fasting where people only eat in the early hours of the morning then start fasting at noon and continue to do so until the early hours of the next morning. The purpose of this is to practice self-discipline for the many physical and mental health benefits of fasting when practiced as a lifestyle and not just as a temporary health plan.

- This is another form of Intermittent Fasting that is not recommended by medical professionals and other health experts to be used as a means of weight loss as it can be difficult to adjust to, sometimes starting with an initial shock to the system that can increase fluid retention and fat storage in the body's cells.

Credit for the first use of fasting as a means of health improvement can be given to Hippocrates of Kos, a physician of ancient Greece most famous as the father of modern medicine and for being the inspiration for the Hippocratic Oath. This oath is a pledge that new doctors take before they start their career promising to uphold high ethical standards and never cause any harm to another human being.

One of Hippocrates most commonly assigned treatments was to sip on apple cider vinegar in place of regular food consumption for a few days to a week, depending on the severity of the original illness or discomfort. The theory behind this was that the cause of the original sickness was something foul or tainted the patient consumed that affected he digestive tract and spread throughout the body from there. By not eating until the symptoms cleared, the patient's body was given the opportunity to heal without risk of consuming anything else toxic or fueling the sickness with calories and carbohydrates. The apple cider vinegar fought off starvation and kept the body functioning during the fasting period.

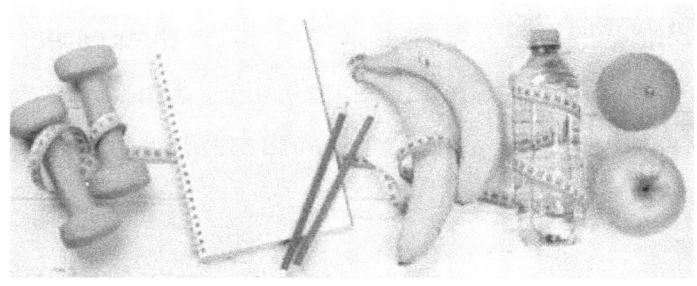

Intermittent Fasting Tip: Apple Cider Vinegar

Apple cider vinegar is still recommended today for detoxing and a number of other positive benefits such as:

- Apple cider vinegar, when regularly consumed, helps to balance pH levels in the body improving digestion, lowering blood sugar numbers and helps to boost energy.
- Apple cider vinegar has also been praised for its effectiveness in fighting cardiovascular disease and improving overall heart health.
- Apple cider vinegar is full of natural antioxidants that can help to fight basic illness such as the common cold and even help to strengthen the body's immune system to fight sickness year-round.
- **For Women:** Apple cider vinegar has a high level of calcium and has been proven to help with strengthening the body's bones and joints. This is one reason it is recommended for women who tend to have greater issues with

skeletal degeneration over time than males do.

- Many doctors and dieticians recommend female patients consume one or two tablespoons of apple cider vinegar per day, diluted in water or undiluted depending on personal preference. Whether or not a woman decides to start fasting or go with a particular diet program, regular apple cider vinegar consumption for the purpose of increasing calcium levels is still a good habit to pick up.

Another theory for why the apple cider vinegar diet and fasting plan was (and is still) so effective is that avoiding food when feeling under the weather is a natural instinctive response anyway. This is one reason people tend to avoid heavy meals and gravitate towards hot tea and broth-based soups when they are not feeling well. This is another reason it works well when paired with lighter and liquid-based diets.

The Science of Intermittent Fasting: How Does It Work?

The human body has two main settings that determine how efficient, powerfully and smoothly our internal systems run. They help to boost energy throughout the day and provide extra fuel from stored fat cells to injured areas to help speed the healing process.

#1 Store Fat for Later Use: When people consume carbohydrates, sugars, and excess protein, the body digests it and uses it for the energy and nutrition it needs now, then transfers the remainder to the liver where it is converted into glycogen to be stored in fat deposits around the body in case of emergency. This is the process most active in the human body during feeding or feasting windows when food is being consumed regularly. When humans eat, the insulin production levels of the body increase thanks to the consumed sugars being digested and deposited in the liver as fat cells. When the liver itself can't hold any more fat but the human continues to eat, all new fat created from ingested food travels to other storage areas such as the core and thighs.

#2 Burn Stored Fat for Extra Fuel: This process is the one most active in times of fasting. Instead of relying on glucose delivered from food sources, the body is able to call upon stored fat cells to convert into emergency energy for the internal organs or body processes. This is the body's natural survival defense against starvation and can happen in times of distress such as being lost or at the mercy of harsh weather. It is also a process that can be initiated and controlled without risk of fatality or illness with Intermittent Fasting. It is monitored and upheld by a person's fluctuating glucose levels. When this begins, the body switches from running on empty sugar cells to burning excess fat so it can maintain energy until individual eats again.

Intermittent Fasting works by creating (and sticking to) a fasting schedule designed to control when the body slips in and out of these processes to minimize fat storage and maximize fat burning.

Intermittent Fasting Tip: Fasting Is Habit & Determination, Not A Miracle Cure

Intermittent Fasting works as a valuable weight loss and health improvement tool only when it is done properly. This means taking the time to make a plan (something the guide will cover in the next chapter) and that means accepting that Intermittent Fasting is not something that is recommended for use in short bursts. There are those that will argue that the term "intermittent" encourages short-term use, however, in the case of Intermittent Fasting, this term is referring to the shorter fasting windows spread throughout each week of fasting, not how long an individual is deciding to fast. For example, someone takes part in one or two weeks of fasting to reach a certain weight loss goal and then abandons their fasting schedule. Typically, what happens is next is that the individual returns to their pre-fasting lifestyle and the weight comes back because the body starts to refill those burned off fat stores it lost during the fasting windows.

Intermittent Fasting is most effective and beneficial when it is undertaken as a lifestyle change. This is particularly true for those with pre-existing health conditions that are related to or can be affected by how the body changes with periods of fluctuating food consumption and deprivation. Not only does adapting Intermittent Fasting into one's daily lifestyle build it as a habit, but it also gives the body some sense of schedule and consistency. Remaining firm in a personalized Intermittent Fasting schedule also gives fasters a greater opportunity to ensure they not only receive but continue to enjoy all of the health benefits fasting can provide.

Why Try Intermittent Fasting?

The uses for and benefits of Intermittent Fasting are numerous and varied. It is important to remember that everyone who tries Intermittent Fasting will have a unique experience as no body responds to controlled fasting.

Intermittent Fasting Tip: Keep It Up!

There will be times when sticking to a fasting plan is challenging and demanding and sliding back into bad habits is bound to happen from time to time. The key to overcoming this when it happens is to never let the negative thoughts that tend to come with trip ups be what holds you down. It is often said that the mind is every person's own worst enemy, it's the most trying times in life that test the actuality of this statement. Not giving up is the only way to go! Keep moving forward, even after stumbling! As long as forward motion is being made then positive progress is being made.

It is also important to remember that speaking with a medical professional, personal physician, dietician or nutritionist before starting any new health programs or when any negative side effects start to show up. Medical professionals are the best option as they can take a look at personal medical history and help with designing a plan or make recommendations for fasting or other health programs based on existing conditions, medical history, genetic risks and questions their patients come in with.

Chapter 2: Intermittent Fasting for Women & Choosing the Right Plan for You

Now that the basics of Intermittent Fasting as a health enhancement option have been laid out, this guide is going to cover the specifics of Intermittent Fasting as it relates to women and their personal health. As women who have been working out or dieting throughout the course of their lives know, not every program that guarantees progress for men will work for females following the same steps, routine or health menu.

In this chapter, we'll take a look at some of the differences in Intermittent Fasting between male and female participants, introduce the first of our simple steps to mastering

Intermittent fasting for women, and provide some helpful tips and tricks to getting started on your own Intermittent Fasting journey!

Intermittent Fasting & The Female Form

There are a number of factors from the biological to the hormonal that can affect the success of a dieting, nutrition or fitness program for women. Some of the negative risks and effects that women see more than men do when starting a new Intermittent Fasting routine include:

- **Hormonal imbalance-** Hormonal imbalances in women can evolve into a wide variety of more serious concerns related to biology and genetics. Some of these concerns include irregular menstruation (length of period or strength of flow) or changes in skin tone and sudden, difficult to clear blemishes.

- **Excessive fatigue-** Fatigue and muscle weakness are two common side effects that come with severely cutting calorie intake, but these are increased for women as the female body relies more on glucose and fat storage to function. While over time the negative side effects decrease or even disappear, the initial transition and adapting to a fasting schedule (depending also on how intense the fasting plan is) is typically more difficult in the first few weeks.
- **Emotional instability-** Also often related to fluctuating hormones, mood swings are a common problem reported by women following an Intermittent Fasting plan, especially in the first two weeks to one month.

It's not all health concerns and difficulties! There are lots of ways that women can benefit from adding an Intermittent Fasting schedule into their daily routine and developing it into their lifestyle in order to help enhance their overall health.

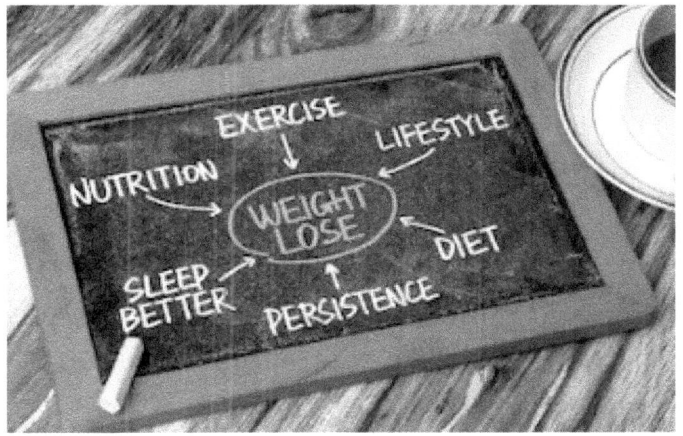

How Does Intermittent Fasting Benefit Women?

Intermittent Fasting is one way that has been shown to assist women with high cholesterol levels, existing heart conditions or heavy risk of heart disease with working on improving their numbers and health options (along with the help of a personal physician or medical professional). This is just one of many health benefits women who have adopted Intermittent Fasting into their daily lifestyle have reported and praised.

Other widely reported positive health effects include:

- Lower risk for the development of and effective treatment of chronic diseases
- Reduced risk of and assistance with controlling obesity
- Women have shown more positive results in the treatment of Type 2 Diabetes and other blood sugar-related conditions with Intermittent Fasting thanks to the increased insulin production the body experiences
- Reduced inflammation throughout the body for those with chronic diseases, lower blood pressure and greater

- control over blood pressure-related conditions
- Intermittent Fasting has proven to be one of the most effective ways for women having trouble getting rid of stubborn fat deposits to finally burn them off, particularly in places like the core and thighs

Women going through menopause have reported Intermittent Fasting as playing a major role in their losing extra weight gained with their hormonal fluctuations. Others have reported seeing more positive stability in their emotional states and the ability to control their emotional impulses throughout the day. The full effects are still being studied on human participants, but in the last decade, tests featuring the effects of Intermittent Fasting on female rats in their menopausal stage have shown encouraging results leading to Intermittent Fasting being more widely recommended for women who are struggling with controlling their menopause symptoms.

While the health benefits of Intermittent Fasting for women specifically are promising, they are still being studied and it is important to remember that everyone's experience with fasting will be different thanks to the personal health factors, biological factors, lifestyle and diet factors, along with any other number of variables that can affect the effectiveness of fasting for individuals.

How Is Intermittent Fasting Riskier for Women?

Female participants in studies across the globe and those reporting their personal results on social media or within fitness communities report many of the same negative effects felt by men throughout the course of adjusting to a new Intermittent Fasting plan. Some of these side effects include:

- Initial hunger pangs and dehydration
- Difficulty concentrating or gaining focus throughout the day
- Headaches, muscle weakness, initial loss in muscle tone

There are some effects that women have experienced and should be watched out for, especially those with a history of trouble or concerns with their menstrual cycles. One such negative effect reported is infertility after long periods of time on an Intermittent Fasting plan. This tends to happen more in women who see a dramatic loss in body fat, especially in the first few weeks (or during the adjustment time).

- In most women, this is nothing to be permanently concerned about as typically periods return to normal and fertility increases in the weeks after

> stopping an Intermittent Fasting plan, particularly for weight loss reasons
- Most wellness experts and medical professionals recommend that women who may be pregnant, are pregnant or are hoping to become pregnant in the near future avoid starting or cease their Intermittent Fasting plan in order to ensure they are in peak condition for childbearing or do not minimize their chances of conceiving

However, for those worried about starting an Intermittent Fasting routine, it is important to point out that even though fasting is still being studied around the world for its long-term benefits and risks on nearly anyone who could ever be interested in trying it (different ages, genders, races, cultural diets, health histories), health and wellness experts all over have written and spoken about its safety, its benefits and its promising progress for men and women alike. It all comes down to being prepared, having all the right information and making a plan that will work and can be stuck with for the long run.

Step One: Making A Plan That Will Get Results

The most significant fact to remember when it comes to getting started with an Intermittent Fasting routine is that the best results come from creating a long-term plan. Fasting is not designed to be used as a means of overnight or short-term weight loss. This is one way that eating disorders develop. There is a difference between fasting and starving. There is a difference between intentionally avoiding food in search of some kind of miracle cure and Intermittent Fasting as a lifestyle change. It is also crucial to remember that it is best to speak with a medical professional before making any kind of major change that could affect your personal health.

Gather All the Information You Can

Creating a plan is the perfect way for first-time fasters and anyone curious about the trying Intermittent Fasting to get a good idea of how their body will react to longer fasting windows without worrying about negative side effects like excess fatigue that can come with an abrupt switch to the program. This is particularly true for those who have decided not to ease themselves in by cutting back on one meal or a couple of hundred calories at a time in the weeks preceding their first official fasting window.

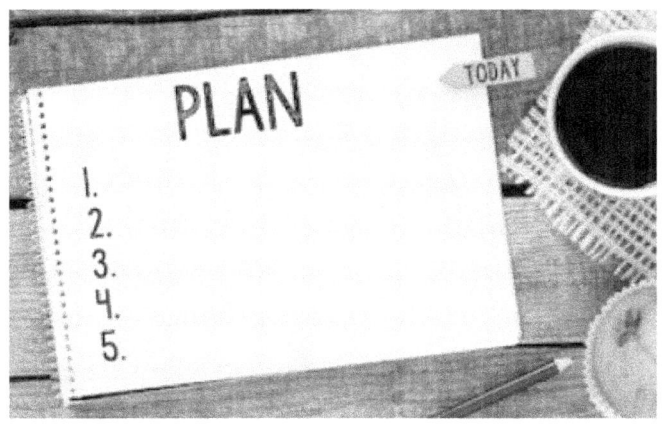

Before planning your first major fasting window or initiating an Intermittent Fasting plan, find out all of the information you can on fasting, on fitness, on diets that work with fasting schedules to maximize health benefits and any other questions that may be causing concern, hesitation or just remain unanswered. The more information you have in at your personal disposal, the easier it will be to create a plan you can stick to that will also deliver the most health benefits with the least side effects.

Determine Your Motivation & Set Realistic Goals

Before you start any kind of diet or fitness routine, it is important to understand why you are wanting to undertake the change and all that comes with it. Just because a new health trend is taking the world by storm, it does not mean that it is the best option for everyone or that it will work for everyone. Any kind of diet or fitness routine requires adaptability, focus, determination, and sacrifice. This is one reason why it is a good idea to determine, if not write out, your motivations for wanting to start an Intermittent Fasting routine. Not only will this help with setting goals, but it will also provide a good means of support and motivation on days when temptation comes calling or there's been a trip up in your plans that interrupted your fasting schedule.

Once you know why you want to try Intermittent Fasting, it comes the time to set your health goals and expectations for the schedule you're planning to start. Where do you want to be in one month, three months, six months and a year? Even if you are unsure about how quickly your body will adapt to Intermittent Fasting along with any other programs you may be trying with it (such as a specific diet or exercise routine), setting goals before you begin your Intermittent Fasting plan gives you a starting place for goals and progress when it comes the time to make adjustments to your schedule.

One step new faster can take to ease their planning and preparation stages is making a list of questions they have and then taking to the internet, to their local gym or to any healthcare professional seeking the answers they need to start moving forward.

Asking the Right Questions

When creating a fasting schedule, there are a number of questions to ask yourself before starting, such as:

- What are my short-term health goals (three to six months) and long-term health goals (one year and beyond)?
    - This could be a certain number of pounds or inches lost with the help of Intermittent Fasting. It could also be less specific fitness-wise such as becoming fit enough to tackle a certain trail in your area or maybe be able to walk a marathon.
- Have I chosen the right Intermittent Fasting method for meeting my personal needs and goals? (Something we will be covering at the end of the chapter.)
- Is fasting the best option for me?

- Have I spoken with my personal physician or other medical professional to ensure a safe transition into and consistency with Intermittent Fasting in the long-term?
- Is the plan I've laid out realistic for my current health status and existing conditions, as well as for reaching my personal health goals?
- Have I weighed the benefits versus the risks of starting an Intermittent Fasting plan and determined what I can do to make the transition as easy as possible before starting?

As soon as these questions are fully answered, each person has what they need to take their first steps toward success with an Intermittent Fasting lifestyle.

The Importance of Designing A Realistic Fasting Plan for Your Lifestyle

One of the things people fall in love with when it comes to Intermittent Fasting is how adaptable it is to almost any kind of daily schedule. With a variety of popular methods that range in time frames, calorie intake or the number of days they last, anyone can find a fasting schedule that works for them. This is a key part of laying out a personalized Intermittent Fasting plan: find a fasting method with a schedule that will work with your existing daily schedule on a longer basis than one or two weeks. Choosing a schedule that you can stick to is fundamental in finding success with Intermittent Fasting.

Intermittent Fasting Tip: The Best First Step Is the Baby Step

This is true for any kind of major lifestyle, diet or fitness change. Sudden changes can send the body into episodes of mild shock that can either clear up with time and determination or escalate into lager health concerns.

The best way to start fasting (particularly for those who have never attempted it or attempted it without success before) is to ease your body into by restricting daily calorie consumption and skipping a meal every day for a week. This makes it less of a shock to the system and the body can take its time adjusting to switching between fat storing and fat burning processes smoothly and without upsetting the digestive system.

Once you've seen how the body reacts to skipping a meal and reducing calorie intake, then you can take another step by reducing by another hundred calories a day or by eating lighter meals for the ones you aren't skipping. In addition to softening the reaction in the body, minimizing calorie intake before beginning a long-term fasting routine helps with mentally preparing oneself and feeling more in control of new habits and challenges that everyone faces at the start of a new health program.

From Method to Mastering: The Different Types of Intermittent Fasting

One of the reasons so many people around the world are seeing such explosive success with Intermittent Fasting is that there are a variety of methods that have been developed through study and experience to meet a range of health desires and achieve any number of personal wellness goals. In this section, the guide will give readers a closer look at the most popular, studied and proven to be an effective method of Intermittent Fasting, how they work and who they work best for.

The 16/8 Method: A Popular Choice for Busy Adults & Beginners

This plan creates feeding and a fasting window each day, splitting it into 16 hours of fasting and 8 hours of normal feeding in order to maximize their fasting benefits and adapt to a schedule on a daily basis. The simplest way to master this method of Intermittent Fasting is for the faster to set their feeding window to start around noon or lunchtime each day, skipping breakfast and automatically reducing their daily calorie intake by at least a quarter, maybe by a third. The feeding window would end just before bedtime for most people, which works out as most nutritionists and dieticians recommend not eating in the hours before bed and in the later hours of the evening.

This time table may not work for everyone, so it is important to point out that the hours themselves are not critical as long as they fit with a person's daily schedule in a way that supports their energy needs instead of causing hunger and fatigue during peak physical or mental activity. As long as the fasting windows themselves are kept to, all excess binging is avoided during feeding windows and the schedule is one that can be maintained with their lifestyle, then this method of Intermittent Fasting should yield positive results for those who choose this one as their fasting plan of preference.

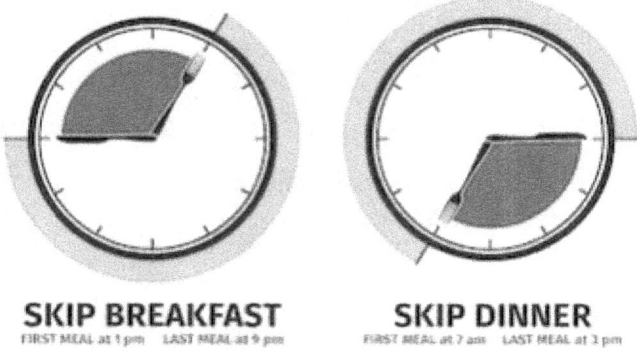

The chart above shows two of the most popular daily fasting and feeding windows for those following this method of Intermittent Fasting to their own advantage.

For women who choose this method, the shorter fasting window of 8 hours and longer feeding window of 16 hours to begin with one or two days a week as a way to adapt your body to the effects of fasting can deliver better results with fewer negative side effects in the early weeks of a new schedule. For those who are concerned about the effects of consistent longer fasting windows on the female form, there are other methods more commonly recommended for women interested in fasting.

Alternate Your Fasting Schedule or Fast Every Other Day: A Universally Balanced Method of Intermittent Fasting

When properly balanced, men and women alike can benefit from this style of Intermittent Fasting, but it is only recommended for experienced fasters when used for health enhancement purposes. Other groups of people that employ this method of Intermittent Fasting are those using fasting as a means of strengthening their spiritual self or coming closer to their individual deity. It requires a higher level of devotion, restriction, and discipline than other methods of Intermittent Fasting and can easily become demanding and overwhelming.

Most commonly called the Alternate Day method, this version of Intermittent Fasting involves the participant eliminating all calorie consumption (even in liquid form) for three or four non-consecutive 24-hour fasting windows each week, eating normally or following a diet with a restricted calorie count on the remaining (or refueling) days. While this method delivers faster, more noticeable results more often than other Intermittent Fasting methods, it also is usually the one complained about the most for initial negative side effects and difficulty to follow for extended periods of time.

This is another method that can work for female and male fasters but is not recommended for women as their first choice for a fasting plan. This is particularly true for women who are at the age where they are most fertile and those who are pregnant, could become pregnant or are trying to become pregnant as this method of Intermittent Fasting has the most potential to negatively affect fertility levels and regular menstruation in women participants.

An Ideal Option for Women of All Ages: The 5/2 Intermittent Fasting Plan

At its core, the 5/2 Intermittent Fasting method is a simplified version of the Alternate Day method, designed for newcomers to fasting, those who have has difficulty with more intensive fasting programs and those who are looking to get the most out of their Intermittent Fasting routine. This method is also the most recommended for women of all ages as the refueling and feeding windows are much more adept to encouraging health benefits such as weight loss and fat burning, while they are less likely to have an effect on menstrual cycles and hormone levels.

With this method of Intermittent Fasting, participants do not completely eliminate their daily calorie intake during fasting times, but instead, they reduce their calorie consumption to a small percentage (30-50%) of what they consume on their average feeding days. This is a good method to employ for those who want to try a more intense form of fasting but want to ease their body into it. To begin this plan properly, two non-consecutive days out of the week the faster would consume around 500 or 600 calories as their fasting day and then eat per their regular calorie consumption the remaining five days each week.

When the body adjusts to this method, those who are ready to increase their fasting windows for enhanced health benefits or extended results can switch to a 4/3 Intermittent Fasting schedule. They would still consume only a small amount of their daily calorie intake on fasting days instead of avoiding them completely. This method is the best for women as their body never has to worry about operating solely on stored fat deposits but is encouraged to do so without increasing the amount of fat stored during feeding windows or on normal eating days.

Once a person has chosen his or her preferred Intermittent Fasting method to meet their personal health goals, the next step is to take the information you've gathered and follow these steps:

- Choose a day to start your Intermittent Fasting plan
- Set your personalized schedule from there for at least the first three to four weeks
    - This will help with meal planning, scheduling events with friends and family, grocery budgeting and so much more!
- Make a list of everything you will need to make sure you have at hand or in your kitchen before your first official Intermittent Fasting window
    - This is something the guide will cover more in-depth in the next chapter

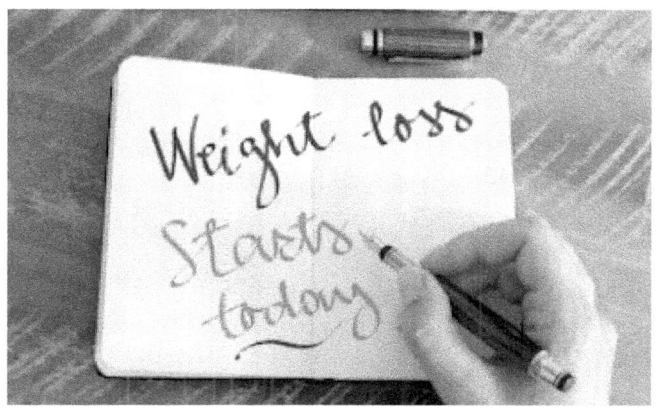

Now that you understand the basics of Intermittent Fasting, how it affects women differently than male fasters, and how to plan the best personalized fasting schedule to meet your needs, keep reading to learn what steps need to be taken to ensure personal success with Intermittent Fasting!

Chapter 3: Setting Yourself Up for Success

Now that we've explored the basics of Intermittent Fasting, how it can be used to improve health conditions and how to choose the right Intermittent Fasting plan to meet personal health goals, let's take a closer look at some steps newcomers to fasting can take in order to increase the chances of success with the program in general and their chosen path specifically. There are easy ways to conquer this popular program to reap the most health benefits and the next two steps in our collection of seven simple steps to mastering Intermittent Fasting as a lifelong health and wellness tool for women!

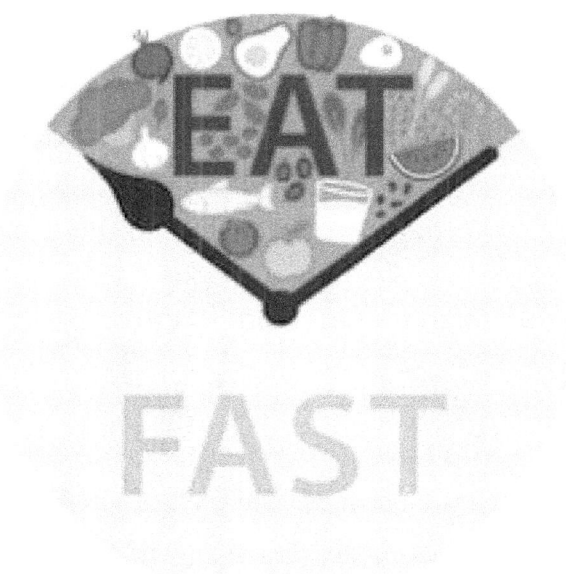

Step Two: Be Prepared Before You Jump Right In!

Adventure can be fun but new habits and routines rarely run smoothly or even get off of the ground without some planning and preparation. This is particularly true for women thanks to the many biological, hormonal, genetic and environmental factors that can affect female participants from seeing the positive results they hope for with Intermittent Fasting. There are ways to counteract these issues when they come up, and in some cases even help prevent them from interfering with forward progression.

Plan Your Exercise Based on How Your Body Feels

Regular exercise is a critical part of maintaining a healthy figure and lifestyle. However, starting an Intermittent Fasting routine can take a toll on the body in the early days and it is often recommended that new fasters not completely stop exercising until they see how their body responds, but to scale it back or at least make sure not to push themselves further than average until they have had the proper time to adjust to the physical, mental and emotional changes that come with a serious alteration to daily routine.

Experts and long-time fasting participants recommend that newcomers focus their exercise times when the body seems to have the most energy to spend on physical activity without leaving the faster fatigued during work, school or other daily obligations and interfering with the course of their daily lives. It is not recommended that exercise stop completely in the early days of Intermittent Fasting as fatigue can overwhelm the body as muscle weakness and other negative side effects make themselves apparent. Even if you just get up and stretch throughout the day, take a small walk, nothing too intense, just enough to get the heart pumping and the body moving.

Intermittent Fasting Tip: Keep a Record of Your Personal Experience

It is always better to caution on the side of safety when it comes to making major habitual changes that could potentially affect or bring attention to existing health conditions. Keeping a health diary or some record of how you're feeling as you start your personal Intermittent Fasting plan can be helpful for a number of reasons including:

- Creating a list of symptoms, when they started, how long they lasted and their intensity
- Providing a solid account of happenings, events, obstacles and other circumstances that may have affected the Intermittent Fasting schedule
- Serving as a reminder of all the progress that has been made throughout your Intermittent Fasting journey on days where it may be difficult to stay determined and focused on your health goals

A personal journal will also come in handy when the time comes to make changes to your personalized fasting schedule in order to minimize side effects or increase the challenge when the body has adapted to the current plan and has slowed or ceased forward progress. This can happen over time making it seem as though Intermittent Fasting has become ineffective. The truth is that like with any diet or fitness program, the body learns to adjust to the fasting process and can become immune to its more aggressive effects like weight loss and fat burning. For those who have reached their health goals, there may not be a need to intensify their personalized Intermittent Fasting routine as long as health levels are being maintained and all positive progress has stuck, not started to reverse.

It's all a matter of personal preference and planning, not everyone will need to make major changes to their fasting plan but having a record of your experiences will help along the line. It doesn't need to be each day; it can be a collection of anecdotal experiences only when the symptoms or events are noteworthy like unusual hunger pangs or a severe headache that just wouldn't seem to go away. It should also include the positive events though, such as hitting a certain goal, discovering a new recipe that works within your preferred diet or setting new goals after progress has been made.

Stock Your Kitchen to Support an Intermittent Fasting Routine

Intermittent Fasting is not just about avoiding food. It is also about choosing the right types and amounts of food that are consumed during feeding, feasting or refueling windows (whatever the preferred term for the individual happens to be). It's during these windows where fasters can focus on the type of diet, they want to pair with their Intermittent

Fasting plan to get the most out of their new health and wellness-inspired lifestyle. There is no requirement to change one's eating habits if an individual is content with their current dietary program or if he or she is required due to existing health concerns to stick to a specific type of food consumption.

One of the best parts about Intermittent Fasting that is continuously praised and spoken of in health circles is its ability to be adapted to any existing diet. This means that those with diet-related health conditions such as gluten intolerance or insulin dependency can take part in fasting as a health enhancement tool without threatening their physical health or making matters worse.

There are plenty of diets that can be used alongside Intermittent Fasting to create a well-rounded and thorough wellness program, but most experts recommend adopting a low carbohydrate and high protein diet (such as the Keto Diet). Foods high in carbohydrates are typically higher in sugar as well, and carbohydrates break down into glucose more easily than other food groups. On the other side of the spectrum, foods higher in protein take longer to digest, making the person feel fuller for longer periods of time and are also lower in fats and carbohydrates which makes them less like to be broken down to store as fat deposits instead of being burned off.

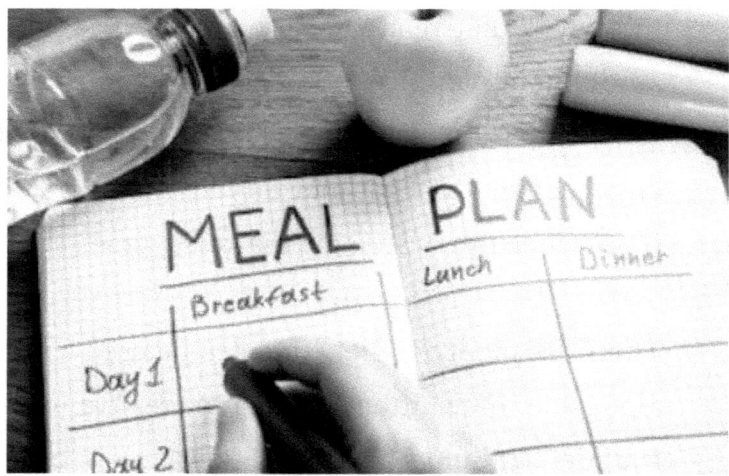

Regardless of the diet you choose, there are steps and actions that can be taken to prepare your kitchen for adjusting to a healthy lifestyle with Intermittent Fasting. Some of these actions include:

- Switching out all processed fats like margarine for healthier cooking oils like coconut oil or olive oil
- Making the switch from refined sugars and sweeteners for healthy alternatives like agave nectar or natural and local honey
- Removing all junk food, sugary drinks and fatty desserts that could damage forward progress via overconsumption of calories
- Replace unhealthy snack options with healthier alternatives like low-carb condiments, snack foods and treats to satisfy a sweet tooth without disturbing a diet or wellness plan

- Fill your cookbooks with low-carb recipes that are as full of flavor as they are health benefits
  - Make sure to find a good collection of healthy snack and dessert recipes that can be made quickly to help on nights when snacking and binging are threatening to throw you off your game

Basically, when it comes to the kitchen: out with the fatty, carb-filled and sugary, in with the organic, local and higher quality meats and produce that promote the health benefits of an Intermittent Fasting lifestyle.

Intermittent Fasting Tip: Sometimes the Gradual Path Is the Best Path to Take

Intermittent Fasting involves adjusting to a new lifestyle that promotes overall health and wellness. For this reason, easing oneself into a personalized Intermittent Fasting plan comes with a number of benefits including:

- A less difficult or troubled adjustment into a particular Intermittent Fasting plan
- More time to monitor how the body is reacting to fasting as a regular part of life so that adjustments can be made to ease discomfort or clear potential negative effects
- An easier time tweaking, fine-tuning and adjusting their individual plan to combat side effects or maximize health benefits

Those who look at fasting as a quick fix to a certain concern or condition will typically see less progress and benefits than those who accept it as a change in lifestyle for the betterment of their overall health and wellness. It is easy to get excited at the start of any new health journey, but with Intermittent Fasting, the more time is taken to understand the feelings and changes the body is communicating, the more likely a person is to see long-term success with their personalized (and continuously developing) fasting plan.

Get A Professional Opinion to Guarantee Health & Safety

The best advice to take when it comes to diets, fitness, and fasting is that from a healthcare professional, preferably a personal physician who is already familiar with the participant's personal medical history and current health status. If there isn't a personal physician involved, a dietician or nutritionist can provide medical information about potential risks and offer advice on how to maximize Intermittent Fasting potential as well.

That completes the basics and fundamentals of Intermittent Fasting for women! All that's left is to make your personalized plan and take your first steps toward a healthy lifestyle supported by Intermittent Fasting.

Step Three: Schedule Your First Fasting Plan

Taking the first step of any journey is a fascinating, confusing and exciting action, and Intermittent Fasting is no exception. The good news is that with this guide, you have already begun setting yourself up for success with your personal Intermittent Fasting journey by collecting your information, writing out your goals and motivations, choosing the right fasting schedule for your individual needs, stocking your kitchen with healthy staples, and taking control of your daily fitness routine to help with adjusting to the new fasting and feeding windows.

Plan Out More Than Just One Week at A Time

One of the best ways to set yourself up for success before you even start fasting is to lay out three to four weeks of fasting and feeding windows at a time. Many find that having a calendar, chart or other kinds of visual representation of their Intermittent Fasting routine helps with things like:

- Keeping track of fasting and feeding days
- Keeping track of progress made and when goals are scheduled
- Making plans with friends and family around your Intermittent Fasting schedule or knowing how to prepare or adjust the times in order to fully enjoy your events and meetings with the people you love

- Planning meals, making grocery lists and scheduling fitness windows can also be made easier by creating a schedule that can be seen and referenced whenever need be

Getting into this habit of planning out fasting windows in three to four week blocks ahead of time helps with staying strong, focused and dedicated to a personal Intermittent Fasting schedule in the long-run.

Choosing the Best Day to Start A New Intermittent Fasting Routine

The best day to start any kind of new change that can have an effect on both the physical and mental functions in the body is a day where your schedule is at its easiest and you have at least one day (preferably two days) to rest following it. The main reason for this is that no one person knows for sure how their body is going to react to the fasting plan they have chosen, particularly if this is their first time ever trying Intermittent Fasting or they haven't taken the time to ease themselves into their new fasting plan. Starting a fasting plan on a demanding day at work or another kind of day that requires an individual to be at their physical and mental peak performance is not recommended as fatigue, nausea, hunger, and dehydration are some of the most common side effects reported on the first day of an Intermittent Fasting routine.

Not everyone experiences adverse effects on the first day, sometimes it can take up to a week for the body to respond to the changes that happen when fasting becomes a regular part of a person's daily routine. This is why having at least a couple of days off after one's first fasting window (especially if it is a longer window or also happening at the start of a dietary change) is recommended, particularly for those who are new to Intermittent Fasting.

Many people like to start their Intermittent Fasting schedules on three-day weekends or spring break. Others stay true to the spiritual origins of fasting and start their Intermittent Fasting schedules during holy times such as Lent or Ramadan. It all comes down to personal preference, just make sure to take the time and make a plan before just diving in or you're starting off at a disadvantage.

What to Expect in the First Week on a New Intermittent Fasting Schedule

For those new to Intermittent Fasting, the first week can be the most worrisome and challenging. Knowing what to look out for and how to overcome obstacles that develop in the early days of a new Intermittent Fasting routine can help make the transition painless and enjoyable for those who have done their preparation and planning. This section of the guide will cover practical tips and tricks on what to expect in the first week of a new Intermittent Fasting plan and how to master fasting in no time!

Intermittent Fasting Tip: Drink More Water Than You Were Before You Started Fasting

Dehydration is one of the most common side effects reported by men and women during their first week of a new or altered Intermittent Fasting plan. The main reason for this is that the water weight is the first to go when fasting and fat burning processes take over and the body requires more hydration than before in order to comfortably function and perform. Any negative effects related to hydration can be easily diminished or even avoided by simply ensuring you're consuming six to eight glasses of water a day.

- Pay attention to hunger pangs as in the first week as well. Many times they can be attributed to thirst and dehydration, rather than lack of food consumption.

Another effect many women specifically report within their first week of a new fasting routine is initially some trouble getting to sleep (between the first three and five days on the new fast schedule). The good news is that after that, the largest percentage of people both men and women) practicing Intermittent Fasting as part of their daily lives have experienced deeper periods of sleep and quicker times for falling asleep each night the more time they stuck with their personalized fasting plan.

All new fasting participants can expect to experience symptoms like the following in their first week of Intermittent Fasting:

- Muscle weakness or soreness
- Nausea, constipation and other digestive complications
- Hunger pangs and increased thirst

- A tendency to get easily distracted or have difficulty gaining or maintaining focus

The best way to combat these issues so that they do not interfere with personal health progress is to make sure that even during fasting windows, enough water is being consumed, enough calories are being eaten during feeding windows and the body is not being put under any excessive strain until it has had time to adapt to a fluctuating eating and fasting schedule.

Now that it's all planned out and you're ready to get started, let's take a look at Intermittent Fasting as a lifestyle change and taking the plunge for long-term health and happiness!

Chapter 4: Taking Your First Intermittent Fasting Steps

In this chapter, the guide will provide a sample two-week fasting schedule designed for women using the 5/2 method of Intermittent Fasting so that those still curious about how to plan their fasting routines can see how they should look.

Step Four: You Have a Plan... Now Take the Plunge!

By this step in our guide, readers should fully understand Intermittent Fasting, how it works and the science behind it, how the program is different for female participants and they also should have chosen which fasting method they believe will be the most effective and helpful in reaching their personal heath goals.

In the Days Before Your First Fasting Window

One of the most important last steps to take before finally starting a new Intermittent Fasting schedule is to do one final overview of your plan, everything you've prepared and all of the lists you've made to ensure that you have everything you need to get started and continue your fasting experience without interruption.

Also, use this time preceding your first fast to take stock of how you're feeling. Are there any discomforts or health concerns you're experiencing before the fasting has started? These are important to watch going into the first two weeks of a new diet or health program as they can be made worse by new changes in body processes or they can disappear as a benefit of the fasting. It depends on the symptoms, their causes and how they are treated going into the first fasting window.

Intermittent Fasting Tip: Don't Start A New Diet the Same Day You Start A New Fasting Schedule

As we've already discussed, starting an Intermittent Fasting schedule takes a toll on the body. The same can be true of diets, particularly those that are dramatically different from an individual's current eating habits. While diets can be a powerful addition to an Intermittent Fasting routine (especially for those interested in the weight loss and fat burning benefits) they can have their own uncomfortable or negative effects on the body that can be misinterpreted as being caused by the adjustment to a fasting schedule if the two are started at the same time.

If you are interested in beginning a new diet as a part of their new Intermittent Fasting plan, experts and long-time fasters recommend either starting the diet at least two weeks before the first scheduled fast or waiting at least two weeks to a month before starting a new diet after the fasting has started. This ensures the body has time to adjust to whichever changes start first and that the effects of one on the body can be identified for what they are and not mistaken for being caused by another.

First Two Weeks Sample Intermittent Fasting Schedule for Women: The 5/2 Method

The 5/2 Intermittent Fasting method is the one most recommended for women interested in creating a fasting schedule that will help reach their personal health goals without creating too much risk to the menstrual and hormonal processes in the body. With that in mind, this two week sample Intermittent Fasting schedule was designed for beginners and those having trouble laying out a schedule of fasting and feeding windows.

.

Fasting Day One: Your First Fast & How to Go About It On the 5/2 Intermittent Fasting Method

The first day of any fasting routine can be demanding and uncomfortable. Luckily, with the 5/2 method, hunger pangs and dehydration are less likely to occur in the first week as fasting days are not totally free of calorie consumption, but rather just planed around a smaller number of calories to be consumed. With the 5:2 method of Intermittent Fasting, fasters are focused on reducing their calorie intake to 500 or 600 calories (for many this is about 25% of their regular daily food consumption) instead of completely eliminating food on fasting days.

Remember the feeling of accomplishment that comes with completing your first day of fasting. It may seem like a simple victory, but in order to stay motivated when Intermittent Fasting gets discouraging, it's key to your personal success to celebrate each forward step you take throughout your health and wellness adventure with Intermittent Fasting.

Feeding Days Two & Three: Back to Regular Calorie Consumption & Ready for Your Next Fast

Congratulations on completing your first fasting day! You can go back to consuming the number of calories for your chosen diet or the number of calories you are accustomed to in your daily eating habits. While it can be a relief to know that you are not as restricted as you would be with total fasting, it is still critical to your long-term Intermittent Fasting plan to make healthy food choices and avoid overeating if you are still experiencing hunger pangs from your first fasting day the next morning.

Find some time during these regular feeding days in order to reflect on how you are feeling. Can you notice any changes? Are they positive ones?

Intermittent Fasting Tip: Listen to Your Mind & Body Throughout the Course of the Week

Spend the extra non-fasting day of your first week mentally preparing yourself for your next fast (the first fasting window of the next week) and another week of scheduled Intermittent Fasting for your health. This can involve getting out and taking a contemplative walk or maybe taking up meditating. For some, this simply means relaxing and enjoying the victory of surviving their first week of Intermittent

Fasting. Some important questions to ask at the end of the first planned fasting week:

- How am I feeling? Physically, mentally and emotionally?
- Is there anything about the personalized fasting plan I've created that I am certain isn't working at this point?
- Are there any changes I can see that need to be made immediately for my health? Anything that is making me sick or threatening my overall health?
- Are there any symptoms I want to watch carefully over the second week to see if they disappear or if they are signs that an aspect of the Intermittent Fasting plan needs to be changed?

The best way to know whether or not Intermittent Fasting is going to work for you and your ultimate health goals in the long-run is to listen to your mind and body, what they are trying to communicate and how they are reacting when changes are made to diet, eating habits or other health-related factors.

Fasting Day Four: Your Second Fasting Window & The Last One of the First Week

The second fasting window should be easier now that you have some idea of what to expect from how you felt your first fasting day and your reflections over the last two feeding days. Considering it is only the second fasting window or day of severely decreased calorie consumption, it is still understandable that there is still stomach pain, digestive discomfort, muscle, and mental fatigue throughout the day as your body adjusts to not having its regular calorie level.

One thing to concentrate on during this second fasting window are the times when you feel the most fatigued or distracted. Make a note of them on your phone or take some notice of the time whenever you start to feel like you're dragging or losing your determination. Knowing the times when the calorie reduction is affecting your body the most can help with planning out when and what to eat throughout the day in order to prevent fatigue and mental drain from interrupting your daily routine.

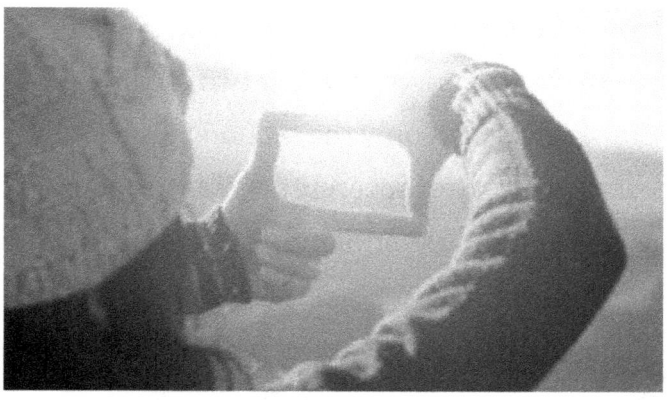

As with the first fasting day (and all of the other fasting days to come), pay attention to how you are feeling physically, mentally and emotionally as any noticeable pain can be a sign of something that needs to be adjusted with your Intermittent Fasting plan. Make sure that you're keeping some kind of record of your symptoms, both positive and negative. These records can be extremely helpful when speaking with medical professionals about fasting or diets, they also provide solid documentation of how exactly Intermittent Fasting is working to help get you to your personal health goals.

Feeding Days Five, Six & Seven: Relax, Reflect & Refuel Before the Start of Your Second Week

Back to eating normally (within reason)! Remember to watch what you're consuming as overeating on your feeding days can back track any forward momentum you should start to make with your personalized Intermittent Fasting routine. There is good news though for those who struggled with wanting to snack throughout their first two fasting windows: most men and women report that they aren't as hungry going into their second week of Intermittent Fasting as they were during their first two fasting windows. It will vary from person to person as it depends entirely on how quickly an individual's body embraces the new calorie consumption and reduction levels.

Take these days to reflect over your first week of Intermittent Fasting and consider what, if any, alterations or changes need to made to the fasting plan you began your first week with. If your negative side effects are not anything troubling, wait until the end of the second week to make any changes. This ensures the body has plenty of time to fix the discomfort itself as part of adjusting to the Intermittent Fasting. However, those who are experiencing anything more than mild stomach discomfort and occasional hunger pangs should put their fasting schedule on hold and speak with a medical professional before continuing.

Fasting Day Eight: One More Hill, Then Nothing but Easy Valleys!

You've reached your third fasting window and third day of severe calorie reduction. Last week you got to see how your body would react to fasting and this week you'll want to continue to watch reactions and listen to how the body is communicating. There is a lot to celebrate going into this fasting window, you've already gotten the first week under your belt and you've held on through two of the most demanding fasting windows anyone who tries Intermittent Fasting will ever experience.

On the other hand, the third day is the fasting window that most people report as being one of the most difficult obstacles in adjusting to Intermittent Fasting. One reason for this is that this is the day many people start to see fasting as a long-term lifestyle change and not just a diet program. This thought can easily become overwhelming, especially for those who are still experiencing negative side effects. Many people find themselves sliding backwards or even being tempted to quit on this third day, but for those who push past their psychological barriers and make it through this window, there is nothing left to hold you back from success with Intermittent Fasting.

Feeding Days Nine & Ten: Keeping an Eye Out for the Subtle Effects

Well done! Another fasting window down and now the body can relax and refuel with healthy food choices filling the daily calorie consumption. By the middle of the second week, many Intermittent Fasting practitioners report that their negative effects are beginning to lighten, if not already completely disappeared.

Now that the painful and sickening symptoms are all but gone, some newcomers to Intermittent Fasting notice that they are more emotional and impulsive in their words and actions. What and when people eat can affect hormones and other mental processes that control speech and behavior. If an individual is experiencing severe mood swings or unusual behavior while adjusting to Intermittent Fasting, it may simply be a temporary effect of adapting to a new fasting routine or it may be a sign that something in their diet or fasting routine needs balancing.

It is also a good idea to try and test your energy limits as your body adapts to all of the new changes and the negative effects disappear. This can help to determine if you should add or reduce energy-focused recipes like power smoothies or protein bowls in your weekly menus.

Fasting Day Eleven: Your Fourth Fasting Window & It's Feeling Like Second Nature by Now

This is your final fasting day in this first two weeks and you should be having no issues with being physically and mentally fatigued or any further digestive discomfort. These are signs that there may be something off balance in your diet or that the fasting schedule you've chosen is not right for your body type. Most experts agree that two weeks should be more than enough time to understand how your body is reacting to your Intermittent Fasting schedule before any changes are made to your original plan.

Feeding Days Twelve, Thirteen & Fourteen: How Far You've Come & Where to Go from Here

Most experts agree that two weeks should be more than enough time to understand how your body is reacting to Intermittent Fasting schedule. At this point in your new fasting plan (by the end of your second week), this is the time to make your alterations, finetuning and major changes. Maybe you've discovered your body isn't reacting to the Intermittent Fasting schedule you've started and you're ready to cut your calories further on your fasting days or try a more intense form of fasting. This could also be a time to adjust your carbohydrate consumption or increase how much protein you're eating on your refueling days.

If you are still struggling with negative side effects by the end of your second week, think about what is causing them and how you can adjust your plan to counteract them. If any existing health problems have gotten worse or new symptoms are appearing that could be a sign of worsening conditions, stop the program immediately and seek medical advice.

Tips & Tricks for Conquering the First Two Weeks of Intermittent Fasting

It may seem daunting, even after all of the time and preparation put in, but Intermittent Fasting has proven to be well worth the initial effort when it is finally mastered! Here is a closer look at some of the most popular and proven advice shared by healthcare experts, fitness communities and experienced fasting participants around the world looking to help others reach their best selves with Intermittent Fasting.

Take a multivitamin or fill your daily calorie consumption with foods full of vitamins and minerals like spinach and other leafy greens. When people suddenly reduce their calorie intake, it is common that for them to also miss out on critical vitamins and minerals the body needs in order to function properly. This can lead to a weakened immune system, lowered mental performance and a number of other symptoms that can easily be mistaken as side effects of the Intermittent Fasting schedule, but can be fixed simply with a daily dose of nutrients or more added into food consumption during feeding windows.

Keep a visual record of your progress with progress pictures! Social media has created a supportive community where people on diets or trying new fitness programs can reach out to others when they have questions or want to share their experiences. One act that has become popular around the world is the taking of progress pictures so that people can show off the benefits they're enjoying, celebrate with others when they reach their goals, or have a visual record of all of their accomplishments to look at and read over on the days Intermittent

Fasting gets difficult. The first progress picture should be taken on the day before or the day of the first fast. This gives the most accurate representation of where the faster started their journey. Some like to take progress pictures weekly or bi-weekly, some wait until they meet each of their set goals. Still, others only take the when there is a noticeable difference, or a dramatic amount of progress has been made so they have a comparison photo to post next to their original progress picture from the beginning of their Intermittent Fasting experience.

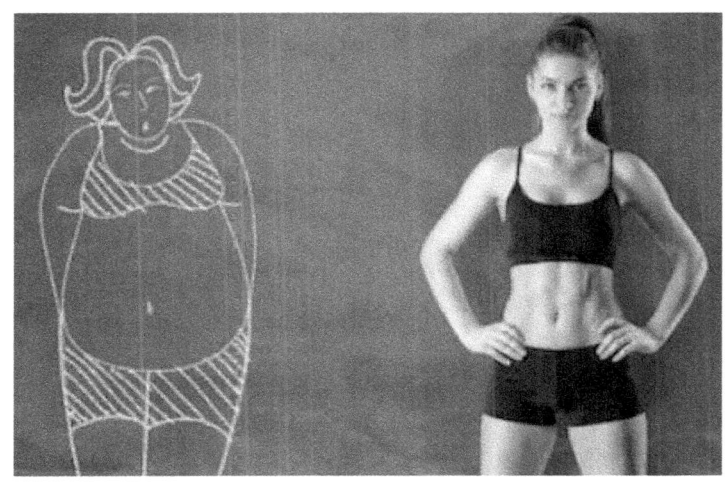

Reach out to your local gyms or health community centers to meet others who are trying Intermittent Fasting, or even just altering their lifestyle in order to improve their overall health. They may not be experts and any advice given should be confirmed with a doctor first, but local dieters, health and fitness enthusiasts are the perfect people to seek out for those looking to build support groups or seeking encouragement during complex obstacles and setbacks. If there aren't any local groups or communities active in your area, social media is a good alternative. Take to Facebook, Twitter or any other site your frequent in search of fellow Intermittent Fasting participants! Intermittent Fasting can be restrictive and can affect social outings if allowed to. Never forget that you're not alone! All you need to do is reach out.

Chapter 5: The Two Week Check-In Point & How It Can Make All the Difference In Successful Intermittent Fasting Plans

Whether you have decided to take your progress pictures weekly or only at major landmarks in your Intermittent Fasting journey, now is the time for another one. Congratulations on passing your first fortnight of Intermittent Fasting! Now it is time for the first bi-weekly fasting plan check-up.

As we have previously discussed in this guide, keeping track of how you are feeling, how your body is responding, and any progress being made is imperative to being successful in the lifestyle change involved with Intermittent

Fasting as a health enhancement option. Experts and fellow fasters across the globe agree that one of the best ways to ensure forward motion is always being made when Intermittent Fasting is being practiced is to regularly check in on one's self.

Step Five: The Two-Week Check In

Two weeks is the length of time most experts and professionals agree the average body needs to adapt to major dietary or fitness changes. Scheduling a personal check-in every two weeks is a good habit to get into, particularly for those who are new to fasting to try and improve their lifestyle.

<u>Important Questions to Ask Before Making Any Major Changes</u>

The biggest part of check-in is asking all the right questions to ensure a thorough job is done and everything is ready to move forward. Here is a look at some of the most important questions to ask when doing a Two-Week Check In:

- How are you feeling physically, mentally and emotionally?
- How has your progress been? Are you on track to meet the goals you've set?
- Can you think of anything you want to change about your current Intermittent Fasting plan?
- Are your current dietary habits working with your current Intermittent Fasting plan?
- Are there any questions or concerns you have after these two weeks that you need to have answered before continuing with another set of fasting windows?

Any other questions you have that concern your body's reaction to fasting, your progress or anything else you can think of can also be added to the list. This check-in is for your benefit, to make certain that Intermittent Fasting and your other health and wellness programs are working to boost your health as they should be. It may seem like a pain to keep track of, but this is a crucial part of maintaining a healthy lifestyle when yours is intertwined with Intermittent Fasting.

Now Is the Time to Make Your First Changes

Only seeing negative effects so far or no progress at all? By the end of the second week, fasters of all levels should be able to identify their negative effects before seeing them fade away. Intermittent Fasting participants at this stage should also be seeing or at least feeling some kind of improvement in their moods, in their stamina and even in their energy levels.

If there are negative side effects persisting into the third and fourth weeks of your fasting plan or that does not seem to be going away with diet and exercise, speak with a medical professional for solid and trustworthy help. If left untreated, symptoms can develop into larger medical concerns. With any diet or health program, it is always best to be safe when it comes to not feeling well.

However, if there are changes that needed to be made such as further cutting calories or adding and additional fasting day to your week in order to inspire some progress. This could also mean altering your current schedule with another Intermittent Fasting method that may work better for your personal needs. It's all a matter of judgement and determination. While it is okay to seek advice from professionals and experienced Intermittent Fasting participants, the final call on whether or not you're ready to increase or alter your fasting schedule comes down to whether or not you feel you're ready.

Now Is the Time to Start a New Diet

This may not be true for everyone as it depends on how an individual is uniquely reacting to their personalized Intermittent Fasting routine. However, studies have shown that for those wanting to increase their progress or their personal challenge, the end of the second week is one of the most effective and promising times to start a new diet plan. The body has had time to adjust, or at least display how it will react to the new fasting schedule, and the individual has had two weeks to get used to fitting Intermittent Fasting into their daily lives.

Intermittent Fasting Tip: Be Certain or Stay Strong!

Just because you can make changes safely at the two-week mark does not necessarily mean that you have to or even need to. If there are any doubts in your mind about whether you should make a specific change to your diet or Intermittent Fasting schedule, then don't make any changes right now. Give your current plan and program another two weeks to see how symptoms or benefits evolve over that time before making any alterations. Always be certain that you are ready to make a change for the betterment of your health or stay strong on the path you've chosen to ensure your body is adapting well to the fasting routine you've set.

For those who are certain they want to take on a diet that will encourage progress with their chosen Intermittent Fasting plan, there are a number of diets on the market that are praised with pairing perfectly. The Keto Diet is one of the most popular options for those wanting to pair an effective diet with their Intermittent Fasting plan. Fasting is one of the two most commonly practiced and safest options for getting the body in and out of ketosis for health enhancement purposes.

The Mediterranean Diet is another that has proven to work well with Intermittent Fasting plans. Women, however, are not always recommended for this diet as they sometimes find themselves having trouble with initial weight gain when trying this program due to the large number of whole grains consumed on this diet.

Before starting any kind of new diet, especially for those with pre-existing health conditions that could be affected by what is or is not being consumed, it is important to speak with a personal physician. They will be able to answer any questions and address any concerns new fasters have about both their preferred diet programs and fasting plans. Like Intermittent Fasting, dietary changes are not meant to be adopted for short lengths of time, but rather as lifestyle changes that are intended to improve your lifelong health.

All Positive Progress Is Forward Progress

Those just beginning of their Intermittent Fasting journey should start small with skipping breakfast for a week or two and adapt from there if they are worried about taking on too much with a full Intermittent Fasting schedule.

Always pay attention to any changes in your body and alter your plan to counteract them by increasing water consumption or making sure you're getting enough protein and vitamins to make it through each day (fasting or feeding). For those looking for additional information, recommendations or want to share their personal fasting stories, there is a massive community of experienced Intermittent Fasting enthusiasts online that are always ready with helpful tips and encouragement at any stage of fasting.

The main thing is to always keep trying and never give up! There will be set backs and there will be difficult days. It's not about whether or not you end up having to temptation or skipping a fasting day. It's about how you bounce back and get back on track when you slip up! Do obstacles and disappointments that occur in your life have the power to make you give up or become discouraged? Or will you dust yourself off when your fall, stand back up and look back toward the future?

Now that you've checked in on your status, determined whether any changes need to be made, made any required changes and are happy with your current Intermittent Fasting plan, it is time to look at next steps and how to maintain fasting as a lifestyle change to encourage the improvement of your personal health.

Chapter 6: Enjoying Your New Lifestyle Bolstered by Intermittent Fasting!

Now that you've got some experience under your belt, it's time to make the most out of your personalized Intermittent Fasting experience to ensure you are reaping the most benefits for your health and wellness. In this final chapter, we will take a look at our final two simple steps to mastering Intermittent Fasting, how to stay true to the plan you've created, how to stay encouraged when everything seems to be working against and where to go from this point forward on your own carefully designed Intermittent Fasting path.

Step Six: Keep It Up & Follow Through

Getting started with Intermittent Fasting (along with other health and wellness programs) presents its own challenges, but once you've developed the habits and have more experience with weaving fasting windows into your personal life, a whole new set of speed bumps awaits. These obstacles are more spread out and may not be as easily predicted, but they are the ones that come with maintaining Intermittent Fasting as a consistent lifestyle.

Keep A Piece of Motivation with You

One way to stay focused and excited about moving forward with a personalized Intermittent Fasting plan is to carry some kind of visual representation of your motivation, inspiration or goals with you wherever you go. This visual is a valuable tool that can serve as a reminder of why you are putting yourself through the bother on difficult days or remind you how far you've come on days when progress may feel slow or as though it has stopped.

For some people, this is their initial progress picture, taken on or before their first fasting window. Some people keep an encouraging note or an event reminder in a locket or on a slip of paper in their wallet. Still, others braid a necklace out of different colored strings to symbolize their dedication to the Intermittent Fasting plan they've created. There are even those who are so encouraged by their progress that they show it in the form of a personalized tattoo! However, you choose to represent your motivations and goals, make it personal and make it easy to keep with you because you never know when temptation or distraction can strike throughout the day.

Intermittent Fasting Tip: Meet Your Goals Before Setting New Ones

Once you start seeing the progress you've made with your Intermittent Fasting plan, it is easy to get energized and thrilled about your victories and want to set new goals. Setting new goals before achieving the ones you've already created for yourself may not seem like that big of a deal, but it can be a debilitating habit to develop for long-term programs like Intermittent Fasting. Celebrating your victories, no matter how small, has a number of benefits including:

- Building self-confidence through congratulations
- Encouraging more progress with positive reinforcement
- Getting your friends, family and other loved ones excited about your taking your health under control

Make Yourself a Motivational Mantra

Mantras are collections of words or phrases that can be used for meditation or stress relief through repetition. They have been used in different belief systems and personal development courses since the early days of higher thought. Using them as a motivational tool makes any challenge you face throughout your life more personal and memorable experience.

Mantras are simple: choosing a word, two or three individual words or a phrase that encourages or inspires you, makes you feel in control when times or tough, or lifts you up when you're feeling down. For the sake of this example, we will use one that works well for focusing and gathering energy during midafternoon mental lulls.

Sturdy. Grounded. Centered.

Now to get the most out of this particular mantra, ideally, the individual would be standing straight backed, with their feet together and their hands flat against one another at chest level in front of them, as if they were the trunk of an ancient tree. Once the mind is clear and the room is quiet, the individual would just need to close their eyes and slowly repeat the mantra as many times as they'd like (typically until they are calmed, focused or once again empowered and ready to tackle any obstacle in their way).

This is just one example. Personal mantras can be focused on weight loss encouragement, better sleep each night, or any other psychological or emotional concern that could be reinforced by some simple repetitious phrase reassurance. Choose a word, three words or a phrase that means something to you personally. That personal connection will make it more effective in helping you conquer your healthcare.

Step Seven: Planning Your Next Move

You've done it! By the time you've finished *Intermittent Fasting for Women: Seven Simple Steps to Understanding & Mastering the Art of Intermittent Fasting*, you should be well on your way to designing your personalized Intermittent Fasting plan, if you haven't already completed your first two weeks on your plan. Regardless of whether you have started on your personal journey or not, you have already taken a huge first step toward taking control of your lifelong health just by downloading our guide.

Now that the world-changing first steps are out of the way though, it seems like the rest of your Intermittent Fasting life is going to be pretty predictable. However, there will always be new challenges to face, new health concerns to address that may require a change in fasting schedule and new goal accomplishments to celebrate. One of the benefits of Intermittent Fasting as a health enhancement program that has made it so popular is that it is easy to build a steady and consistent schedule around fasting windows because they are so adaptable to any standing schedule.

Set New Challenges & Never Stop Climbing

If you've found the method of Intermittent Fasting that works best for your figure, health and personal needs, just make sure you stick with it! Over time, you may notice that progress has started to slow down or has stopped altogether. This is because over time the body adapts to changes in eating habits and fitness adjustments and tarts to slip back into the fat storing habits it relied on before new health and wellness programs were initiated. No need to get discouraged! If this starts to happen, a simple increase in physical activity, further reduction of calories on fasting days or longer fasting windows followed by lighter feeding periods.

Instead of letting yourself get disheartened by the slowing of personal progress, look at these moments as opportunities to shorten deadlines for meeting goals after increasing fasting times, or as the perfect time to try total fasting (instead of severe calorie reduction for those on the 5/2 Intermittent Fasting schedule). Are there any other goals you're still trying to reach? Have you thought about your next goal levels and when you'd like to reach them?

Keep searching the internet, social media and local health communities for new opportunities or developments in research on Intermittent Fasting and how it can be properly used as a powerful health enhancement tool. Never stop asking questions, never stop learning!

Increase or Intensify Your Regular Exercise Routine

Once your body has had plenty of time to adjust to Intermittent Fasting as part of your daily lifestyle, it comes time to focus on altering and intensifying your fitness routine instead of continuously altering your Intermittent Fasting schedule. In addition to fasting and dieting, exercising assists the body in burning stored fat deposits as fuel and strengthening the body's muscles as it goes.

For those not used to daily exercise routines, starting with something low impact like walking around the neighborhood every morning or swimming in the summertime are a great way to get started. For those who already have a set fitness routine, try adding some extra reps or slightly heavier weights to your existing workouts in order to make them more challenging and effective for toning the body.

Continue with Your Two Week Check-Ins for As Long As Your Are Following Your Intermittent Fasting Plan

Always remember that even if you can't feel them immediately or in the form of pain, symptoms of change related to starting a new Intermittent Fasting routine can appear at any time and can take a serious toll on the physical and mental performance. This is why it is so important to always check in on your personal health (physical, mental and emotional) to ensure that you are always performing at your highest possible ability and are not being held back by their Intermittent Fasting plan, instead of being supported by it.

Get yourself into the habit of doing your two week check ins and you will never have to worry about not knowing how long symptoms have been bothering you, how long it has been since a goal was last met, about forgetting how much progress you have made or how long you have been Intermittent Fasting once you have been fasting like an old pro for a while.

Never Stop Searching, Learning & Striving

No matter your personal health goals are, never start to think that you've learned all there is to know. While guides like this one are useful tools in helping women and any other newcomers to Intermittent Fasting understand the specifics, make a plan designed for their personal benefit and master the art of fasting for health enhancement, there are always new studies being performed and their results published showing new discoveries, developments and methods for fasting that may be just what an individual is looking for to maximize the effectiveness of their personalized plan.

Conclusion

Thank you for enjoying *Intermittent Fasting for Women: 7 Simple Steps to Understanding & Mastering the Art of Intermittent Fasting for Women in Every Day Life!* Hopefully, we have achieved our main goal and provided you with all of the information you could ever hope for on Intermittent Fasting and how it affects the female form. By the end of this guide, readers should have the skills they need to not only get started on their own unique Intermittent Fasting journey but be able to do so with confidence in both their fasting schedule and themselves.

Some of the skills featured in the guide that we hope readers find useful include:

- How to choose the right Intermittent Fasting plan to meet specific health goals
- How to plan or alter exercise routines to be most effective throughout a new fasting plan from helping the body adjust in the first few weeks to making changes to their regular fitness routine based on how the body reacts to Intermittent Fasting
- How to stay focused and determined even through the hardest of days of an Intermittent Fasting lifestyle
- How and when are the best ways/times to make changes or alterations to a personalized Intermittent Fasting plan

From here, the next step is to finish gathering your information and get your first Intermittent Fasting plan together! Fasting can be complex, but the more information fasters have, the better the chances for success become for short-term and long-term health goals. There is not any major hurry to get started with Intermittent Fasting as it is meant to be employed as a lifestyle change, or essentially a lifelong practice that can be:

- Developed based on an individual's current health, wellness, dietary and fitness needs
- Adjusted based on health changes over the years
- Put on pause for necessary circumstances like pregnancy for women or any kind of illness that could be enflamed, rather than helped, by Intermittent Fasting
- Even picked back up again without much frustration or concern when the participant is ready to do so

Don't forget that the purpose of this guide is to provide information, practical steps to follow and advice on how to master the fundamentals of Intermittent Fasting based on research and experience collected and shared on the topic. It is not meant to be used as a medical reference or as a sole source of Intermittent Fasting knowledge, particularly for those with existing health conditions that could be affected by what and how much they are or are not eating on a daily basis. Before starting any kind of major change to personal health plans, diets or fitness routines, it is always not only a good idea, but a critical first step in achieving success through Intermittent Fasting.

Now that you've learned the basics about Intermittent Fasting, what it is and how it works, we sincerely hope that you will be able to use it as a valuable support tool and regular lifestyle practice that will help with not only taking control of your personal health but also maintaining it throughout the course of your life to become and enjoy being a healthier, happier version of yourself! Thank you again for purchasing *Intermittent Fasting for*

Women: 7 Simple Steps to Understanding & Mastering the Art of Intermittent Fasting for Women in Every Day Life!

good luck on every step of your personal health journey!

www.ingramcontent.com/pod-product-compliance
Lightning Source LLC
Chambersburg PA
CBHW071717020426
42333CB00017B/2302